MANAGING DIABETES:

A COMPREHENSIVE SELF HELP BOOK FOR PEOPLE WITH DIABETES.

NATHAN I JOSHUA

Table of content

INTRODUCTION

"Managing Diabetes: A Comprehensive Self Help Book for People with Diabetes" is a guidebook for individuals living with diabetes. The book aims to educate and empower people with diabetes to take control of their condition by providing information on various aspects of diabetes management, including diet, exercise, medication, and blood sugar monitoring. Additionally, the book also cover psychological and emotional aspects of living with diabetes, as well as offer advice on how to work effectively with healthcare providers. The overall goal of the book is to help people with diabetes live healthy, fulfilling lives.

The book provide practical tips and strategies for managing diabetes, such as meal planning, shopping for healthy foods, and coping with stress. It also address common complications of diabetes such as heart disease, nerve damage, and eye problems. Additionally, the book include success stories from people with diabetes, to provide encouragement and inspiration. The information and advice provided in the book is intended to complement the guidance and treatment provided by a healthcare provider. By using this self-help book, people with diabetes can take an active role in their own care and improve their overall quality of life.

Understanding Diabetes

There are two main types of diabetes: type 1 and type 2. Type 1 diabetes is an autoimmune disorder in which the body's immune system attacks and destroys the cells that produce insulin, a hormone that regulates blood sugar. Type 2 diabetes is a metabolic disorder in which the body becomes resistant to insulin and is unable to produce enough of it to keep blood sugar levels in check.

Diabetes is a chronic medical condition characterized by high levels of glucose, or sugar, in the blood. Glucose is an important source of energy for the body, but it must be regulated properly to ensure optimal health. In individuals with diabetes, the body is unable to regulate glucose effectively, leading to elevated levels in the blood.

There are two main types of diabetes: type 1 diabetes and type 2 diabetes. Type 1 diabetes is an autoimmune disorder that occurs when the body's immune system attacks and destroys the cells in the pancreas that produce insulin, a hormone that regulates glucose levels in the blood. Type 2 diabetes, on the other hand, occurs when the body becomes resistant to insulin or the pancreas is unable to produce enough insulin to regulate glucose levels.

Both types of diabetes can lead to a range of serious complications, including heart disease, nerve damage, kidney disease, and eye problems.

Managing diabetes involves maintaining stable blood sugar levels through a combination of lifestyle modifications and medical management. This may include following a healthy diet, engaging in regular physical activity, taking medications as prescribed, and monitoring blood sugar levels regularly.

Early diagnosis and effective management of diabetes can help reduce the risk of complications and improve quality of life. It is important for individuals to be aware of the risk factors for diabetes and to seek medical evaluation if they experience symptoms, such as increased thirst, frequent urination, blurred vision, or slow healing of cuts and bruises.

Working with a healthcare team, including a doctor, diabetes educator, and registered dietitian, can help individuals with diabetes effectively manage their condition and reduce the risk of complications. Regular check-ins with healthcare providers, monitoring blood sugar levels, and making lifestyle changes as needed can help ensure success in managing diabetes.

In addition to lifestyle modifications and medical management, there are several other factors that can impact the management of diabetes:

Stress: Stress can cause fluctuations in blood sugar levels and may make it difficult to manage diabetes effectively. Individuals with diabetes can benefit from stress management techniques, such as deep breathing, meditation, or exercise, to help regulate their blood sugar levels.

Sick days: Illnesses, such as the flu or a cold, can cause fluctuations in blood sugar levels and make it more challenging to manage diabetes. It is important for individuals with diabetes to have a sick day plan in place to ensure that their blood sugar levels are managed effectively during these times.

Alcohol consumption: Alcohol can cause fluctuations in blood sugar levels and may interfere with the effectiveness of diabetes medications. Individuals with diabetes should limit their alcohol intake and always check with their healthcare provider before drinking.

Medications: Some medications can impact blood sugar levels and may require adjustments to the diabetes management plan. Individuals with diabetes should discuss all medications they are taking, including over-the-counter medications, with their healthcare provider.

Travel: Traveling can make it more challenging to manage diabetes, as it may be difficult to maintain a regular routine and access healthy food choices. Individuals with diabetes should plan ahead for travel and make arrangements to ensure that their diabetes management needs are met.

By being mindful of these factors and working closely with their healthcare team, individuals with diabetes can effectively manage their condition and reduce the risk of complications. Regular monitoring of blood sugar levels, seeking support from healthcare providers and support groups, and making changes to the diabetes management plan as needed can help ensure success in managing diabetes.

Complications of diabetes

People with uncontrolled or poorly managed diabetes are at risk of developing a number of serious complications. Over time, high blood sugar levels can damage blood vessels and nerves throughout the body, leading to problems in various organ systems.

Cardiovascular disease is a major concern for people with diabetes. They are more likely to develop heart disease, stroke, and peripheral artery disease. Neuropathy, or nerve damage, is another common complication of diabetes, which can cause numbness, tingling, or pain in the feet and hands, as well as digestive problems and sexual dysfunction.

Diabetic Nephropathy is a type of kidney damage that can occur in people with diabetes. It can cause chronic kidney disease and end-stage renal disease, which may require dialysis or kidney transplant. Diabetic retinopathy is a leading cause of blindness and vision loss among people with diabetes. Foot problems such as peripheral neuropathy and reduced circulation can increase the risk of foot injuries and infections.

Additionally, skin conditions such as diabetic dermopathy, necrobiosis lipoidica diabeticorum, and diabetic blisters can develop. People with diabetes are also at increased risk of hearing impairment and cognitive decline, including Alzheimer's disease. Depression is also more common in people with diabetes and can affect their ability to manage the disease.

Prevention and complication management:

To manage and prevent complications of diabetes, the following steps can be taken:

Maintaining good blood sugar control: Regular monitoring of blood sugar levels and taking appropriate measures to keep them within target range is crucial in preventing diabetes complications.

Exercise and healthy eating: Regular physical activity and a balanced diet can help control blood sugar levels and reduce the risk of complications such as heart disease and obesity.

Blood pressure and cholesterol control: High blood pressure and high cholesterol levels increase the risk of heart disease and stroke. Regular monitoring and appropriate management can reduce this risk.

Foot care: People with diabetes are at increased risk of foot problems, such as neuropathy and infections. Regular foot inspections, wearing proper footwear and taking care of the skin can prevent complications.

Eye exams: Regular eye exams are essential for detecting and treating diabetic retinopathy, a condition that can lead to vision loss.

Smoking cessation: Smoking increases the risk of heart disease and stroke. Quitting smoking can reduce this risk.

Medications: Taking prescribed medications as directed, such as blood pressure and cholesterol-lowering drugs, can help prevent and manage diabetes complications.

It is important to work closely with a healthcare provider to develop an individualized plan to manage diabetes and its complications.

The role of diet in managing Diabetes:

Eating a healthy diet is crucial for managing diabetes. The right foods can help keep blood sugar levels in check and prevent complications. A diet that is high in fruits, vegetables, lean proteins, and whole grains is recommended for people with diabetes. It is also important to be mindful of portion sizes and to limit the intake of added sugars, saturated fats, and processed foods.The role of diet in managing diabetes is significant. A healthy diet can help regulate blood sugar levels, control weight, and reduce the risk of heart disease and other diabetes-related complications.

People with diabetes should aim to consume a balanced diet that is rich in nutrients, low in unhealthy fats and added sugars, and includes a variety of fruits, vegetables, whole grains, and lean proteins. It is also important to limit the intake of salt and saturated fats.

Eating regular, balanced meals and snacks throughout the day can help maintain stable blood sugar levels. It is also recommended to limit the consumption of foods high in simple carbohydrates, such as white bread and sugary drinks, as these can cause rapid spikes in blood sugar levels.

For individuals with diabetes, it is recommended to work with a registered dietitian or nutritionist to develop a personalized meal plan that takes into account individual needs and preferences.

In addition to diet, physical activity, medication use, and stress levels can also affect blood sugar levels, so it is important to address all of these factors as part of an overall diabetes management plan.

Understanding Carbohydrates and Blood Sugar:

Carbohydrates are a major source of energy for the body and are found in many foods such as fruits, vegetables, grains, and legumes. When carbohydrates are broken down by the body, they turn Into glucose, which is the main source of fuel for the body's cells. However, when glucose enters the bloodstream, it must be regulated by insulin to prevent blood sugar levels from getting too high. People with diabetes have a harder time regulating blood sugar, and so it's essential to be mindful of the amount and type of carbohydrates they consume.Carbohydrates play a major role in blood sugar regulation in individuals with diabetes. Carbohydrates are broken down into glucose (sugar) in the body, which is then absorbed into the bloodstream and used as energy.

In individuals without diabetes, the hormone insulin helps regulate the amount of glucose in the bloodstream. In individuals with diabetes, the body either doesn't produce enough insulin or is unable to effectively use insulin, leading to elevated levels of glucose in the bloodstream.

To help manage blood sugar levels, it's important for individuals with diabetes to understand the types and amounts of carbohydrates they consume.

There are two main types of carbohydrates: simple and complex. Simple carbohydrates, such as sugar, candy, and soft drinks, are quickly absorbed into the bloodstream and can cause rapid spikes in blood sugar levels. Complex carbohydrates, such as whole grains, fruits, and vegetables, are broken down more slowly and do not cause as rapid of an increase in blood sugar levels.

To manage blood sugar levels, individuals with diabetes should aim to consume a balanced diet that includes a mix of simple and complex carbohydrates. It is also important to monitor portion sizes and to spread carbohydrate intake evenly throughout the day.

In addition to diet, physical activity can also affect blood sugar levels. Regular physical activity can help the body use insulin more effectively, reducing the need for insulin or oral medications, and helping to regulate blood sugar levels.

It is important to work with a healthcare provider and registered dietitian to develop an individualized meal plan and exercise plan to effectively manage blood sugar levels. Regular monitoring of blood sugar levels and frequent check-ins with healthcare providers can help ensure proper management and reduce the risk of complications associated with diabetes.

Carbohydrates play a major role in blood sugar regulation in individuals with diabetes. Carbohydrates are broken down into glucose (sugar) in the body, which is then absorbed into the bloodstream and used as energy.

In individuals without diabetes, the hormone insulin helps regulate the amount of glucose in the bloodstream. In individuals with diabetes, the body either doesn't produce enough insulin or is unable to effectively use insulin, leading to elevated levels of glucose in the bloodstream.

To help manage blood sugar levels, it's important for individuals with diabetes to understand the types and amounts of carbohydrates they consume.

There are two main types of carbohydrates: simple and complex. Simple carbohydrates, such as sugar, candy, and soft drinks, are quickly absorbed into the bloodstream and can cause rapid spikes in blood sugar levels. Complex carbohydrates, such as whole grains, fruits, and vegetables, are broken down more slowly and do not cause as rapid of an increase in blood sugar levels.

To manage blood sugar levels, individuals with diabetes should aim to consume a balanced diet that includes a mix of simple and complex carbohydrates. It is also important to monitor portion sizes and to spread carbohydrate intake evenly throughout the day.

In addition to diet, physical activity can also affect blood sugar levels. Regular physical activity can help the body use insulin more effectively, reducing the need for insulin or oral medications, and helping to regulate blood sugar levels.

It is important to work with a healthcare provider and registered dietitian to develop an individualized meal plan and exercise plan to effectively manage blood sugar levels. Regular monitoring of blood sugar levels and frequent check-ins with healthcare providers can help ensure proper management and reduce the risk of complications associated with diabetes.

Meal Planning and Portion Control:

Meal planning and portion control are essential for managing diabetes. By creating a meal plan and sticking to it, people with diabetes can better control their blood sugar levels. It's also important to be mindful of portion sizes, as eating too much can lead to weight gain and high blood sugar. A registered dietitian or a certified diabetes educator can help create a meal plan that is tailored to your specific needs.

Meal planning and portion control are important components of managing diabetes. A well-planned diet can help regulate blood sugar levels, maintain a healthy weight, and reduce the risk of diabetes-related complications.

When meal planning, individuals with diabetes should aim to include a balance of carbohydrates, protein, and healthy fats at each meal. It is also important to limit the intake of added sugars, saturated fats, and salt.

In terms of portion control, it is important for individuals with diabetes to be mindful of the amounts of food they are consuming, as well as the types of foods they are eating. Consuming large portions of high-carbohydrate foods, such as bread, pasta, or sweets, can cause rapid spikes in blood sugar levels.

To help with portion control, individuals with diabetes can use measuring cups, a food scale, or visual cues, such as a deck of cards, to estimate portion sizes.

In addition to meal planning and portion control, physical activity and stress management are also important components of managing diabetes. Regular physical activity can help regulate blood sugar levels and reduce the risk of diabetes-related complications, while effective stress management can help maintain stable blood sugar levels.

It is important to work with a healthcare provider and registered dietitian to develop a personalized meal plan that takes into account individual needs and preferences. Regular monitoring of blood sugar levels and check-ins with healthcare providers can help ensure that meal planning and portion control strategies are effective in managing diabetes.Aside from meal planning and portion control, there are other strategies that individuals with diabetes can use to manage their condition:

Meal timing: Spreading carbohydrate intake evenly throughout the day can help regulate blood sugar levels. This can be achieved by eating three main meals and one or two snacks per day.

Food preparation: Cooking at home and preparing meals in advance can help ensure that healthy food choices are available and make it easier to control portion sizes.

Food labels: Reading food labels and paying attention to serving sizes, calorie and carbohydrate content, and ingredient list can help individuals with diabetes make informed food choices.

Eating out: Eating at restaurants or ordering takeout can be challenging for individuals with diabetes, as portion sizes can be larger and it may be difficult to determine the content of the food. To make healthier choices when eating out, individuals with diabetes can ask for nutrition information, opt for grilled or baked options instead of fried, and ask for sauce or dressing on the side.

Snacks: Snacking can help regulate blood sugar levels and provide energy between meals. Healthy snack options for individuals with diabetes include fruits, vegetables, nuts, and low-fat dairy products.

By incorporating these strategies into their lifestyle, individuals with diabetes can effectively manage their condition and reduce the risk of complications. It is important to regularly monitor blood sugar levels, seek support from healthcare providers and support groups, and make changes to the meal plan as needed to ensure success in managing diabetes

Shopping for Diabetic-Friendly Foods

Whole grains: Whole wheat bread, quinoa, brown rice, and oatmeal are all excellent choices.

Fruits and vegetables: These are high in fiber, vitamins, and minerals, and can help keep blood sugar levels stable. Some good options include leafy greens, berries, and citrus fruits.

Legumes: Beans, lentils, and peas are all high in fiber and protein, which can help keep blood sugar levels stable.

Lean protein: Chicken, fish, and tofu are all good options for diabetics.

Healthy fats: Foods such as avocados, nuts, and seeds are high in healthy fats and can help keep blood sugar levels stable.

Dairy: Low-fat dairy products such as yogurt, cheese and milk can be a good source of calcium, protein and other nutrients

When you're shopping, it is important to <u>read the nutrition labels and ingredient lists</u> to help you make informed choices. Avoid foods with high sugar and sodium content, and instead, look for low-sugar, low-carb, and high-fiber options.

It's also important to consult with your ethereal provider or a registered dietitian to develop a personalized meal plan that fits your individual needs and dietary restrictions.

s for you and your diabetes.

In addition to the foods mentioned above, there are several other diabetic-friendly foods that you can consider adding to your shopping list:

Nuts and seeds: These are a great source of healthy fats, fiber, and protein. They can help keep blood sugar levels stable and may also reduce the risk of heart disease.

Fish: Fish, particularly fatty fish such as salmon, tuna, and sardines, are high in omega-3 fatty acids, which can help improve heart health.

Eggs: Eggs are a great source of protein and can help keep you feeling full for longer periods of time.

Herbs and spices: These can add flavor to your food without adding extra sugar or sodium. Some options include cinnamon, ginger, and turmeric, which may have anti-inflammatory and blood sugar-lowering properties.

Low-sugar or sugar-free alternatives: For those with diabetes, it's important to limit added sugars in their diet. Instead, you can opt for sugar-free or low sugar options of your favorite foods such as sugar-free jams, jellies, syrups and more.

When shopping for diabetic-friendly foods, it's important to remember that it's not just about what you eat, but also about portion control and balance. Eating a variety of nutrient-dense foods and limiting processed foods can help you control your blood sugar levels and maintain good health.

Diabetic-friendly breakfast recipes

Avocado and Egg Toast:

Mash half an avocado and spread it on a piece of whole-grain toast.

Top with a fried or poached egg and season with salt and pepper.

Greek Yogurt Parfait:

In a jar or bowl, layer Greek yogurt, berries, and a sprinkle of chopped nuts.

Here are a few diabetic-friendly breakfast recipes that you can try:

Avocado and Egg Toast:

Mash half an avocado and spread it on a piece of whole-grain toast.

Top with a fried or poached egg and season with salt and pepper.

Greek Yogurt Parfait:

In a jar or bowl, layer Greek yogurt, berries, and a sprinkle of chopped nuts.

Veggie Omelette:

Whisk 2 eggs and a splash of milk, season with salt and pepper.

Cook diced vegetables such as bell peppers, mushrooms, and onions in a pan with a bit of oil.

Pour the egg mixture over the vegetables and cook until set.

Smoothie bowl:

Blend together frozen berries, a ripe banana, a scoop of Greek yogurt, and a splash of almond milk.

Pour the smoothie into a bowl and top with chopped nuts and seeds.

Egg and cheese muffins:

Preheat the oven to 350°F.

Whisk together 6 eggs and 1/4 cup of milk, season with salt and pepper.

Grease a muffin tin and divide the egg mixture evenly among the cups.

Top with shredded cheese, diced vegetables or meat, and bake for 20-25 minutes.

These are just a few examples of delicious and diabetic-friendly breakfast options that you can try. Keep in mind that it's important to consult with your ethereal provider or a registered dietitian to ensure that any recipe you choose is appropriate for your specific dietary needs and restrictions.

Tips on eating a diabetic-friendly breakfast

Include protein: Starting your day with a source of protein can help keep you feeling full for longer periods of time and can also help stabilize blood sugar levels. Some good options include eggs, Greek yogurt, cottage cheese, and protein shakes.

Focus on fiber: Foods high in fiber can help slow the absorption of carbohydrates, which can help keep blood sugar levels stable. Whole grains, fruits, vegetables, and legumes are all good sources of fiber.

Watch your portion sizes: It's important to be mindful of the portion sizes of the foods you eat, especially when it comes to carbohydrates. Eating too many carbohydrates at once can cause a spike in blood sugar levels.

Plan ahead: If you're short on time in the morning, consider prepping breakfast the night before. You can make overnight oats, smoothie packs, or even hard-boil eggs to have on hand.

Be mindful of added sugars: Many breakfast foods, such as cereal, granola bars, and yogurt, can be high in added sugars. Be sure to read the nutrition labels and ingredient lists to ensure that you're not consuming too much sugar.

Consult with a professional

Remember to consult with your ethereal provider or a registered dietitian to ensure that your breakfast choices are appropriate for your individual needs and dietary restrictions. They can also help you create a personalized meal plan that works for you.

By following these tips, you can ensure that your breakfast is both delicious and diabetic-friendly, and that it can help keep your blood sugar levels stable throughout the day.

Diabetic-friendly appetizer and snack ideas

Veggie sticks: Cut up a variety of vegetables such as carrots, cucumbers, bell peppers, and celery, and serve them with a low-fat dip such as hummus or Greek yogurt.

Cheese and whole grain crackers: Choose a low-fat cheese such as mozzarella or feta, and pair it with whole grain crackers for a satisfying snack.

Guacamole and salsa with veggies or whole-grain chips: Guacamole and salsa are both low in carbohydrates and high in fiber and healthy fats. Serve them with a variety of veggies or whole-grain chips.

Greek yogurt and berries: Greek yogurt is a great source of protein, and berries are high in fiber. Mix them together for a healthy and delicious snack.

Edamame: Edamame is a type of soybean that is high in protein and fiber and low in carbohydrates. It's a great snack option for diabetics.

Nuts and seeds: Nuts and seeds are a good source of healthy fats and protein, which can help keep blood sugar levels stable.

Hard-boiled eggs: Eggs are a good source of protein and can help keep you feeling full for longer periods of time.

It's important to keep in mind that portion control is key when it comes to snacking and appetizers, as well as to consult with your ethereal provider or a registered dietitian to ensure that the snacks you choose are appropriate for your individual needs and dietary restrictions.

Here are a few diabetic-friendly soup and salad ideas:

Vegetable soup: A vegetable soup made with a variety of low-carb vegetables such as broccoli, cauliflower, and green beans is a great option for diabetics. Avoid adding potatoes, corn, or other high-carb vegetables.

Chicken or turkey chili: Chili made with lean protein such as chicken or turkey, and a variety of low-carb vegetables like bell peppers, onions, and tomatoes is a good option for diabetics.

Greek salad: A Greek salad made with a variety of vegetables such as cucumbers, tomatoes, and bell peppers, paired with feta cheese, and dressed with olive oil and lemon juice is a great option for diabetics.

Caesar salad: A Caesar salad made with a variety of greens such as romaine lettuce, and paired with lean protein such as chicken or shrimp, and dressed with a low-fat Caesar dressing is a good option for diabetics.

Broccoli and cheddar soup: A broccoli and cheddar soup made with low-fat milk and cheese, and paired with a variety of vegetables such as broccoli, cauliflower, and leeks is a good option for diabetics.

Spinach salad: A spinach salad made with a variety of greens such as spinach, paired with lean protein such as chicken or shrimp, and dressed with a low-fat vinaigrette is a good option for diabetics.

It's important to be mindful of portion control and to consult with a ethereal provider or a registered dietitian to ensure that the soups and salads you choose are appropriate for your individual health.

Diabetic-friendly main dish ideas:

Stir-fry: A stir-fry made with lean protein such as chicken, shrimp, or tofu, and a variety of low-carb vegetables such as bell peppers, onions, and broccoli is a good option for diabetics.

Meatloaf: Meatloaf made with lean ground beef or turkey and mixed with vegetables such as diced carrots and zucchini is a good option for diabetics.

Baked or grilled salmon: Salmon is a great source of omega-3 fatty acids, which can help improve heart health. It can be seasoned with herbs and spices and served with a variety of low-carb vegetables such as asparagus or green beans.

Grilled or roasted chicken or turkey breast: Chicken or turkey breast is a great source of lean protein and can be seasoned with herbs and spices, and served with a variety of low-carb vegetables such as Brussels sprouts or green beans.

Grilled or roasted vegetables: Roasted or grilled vegetables such as bell peppers, eggplant, and zucchini can be a delicious and healthy main dish. They can be seasoned with herbs and spices and served with a side of protein such as grilled chicken or fish.

As always, it's important to be mindful of portion control and to consult with a ethereal provider or a registered dietitian to ensure that the main dishes you choose are appropriate for your individual needs and dietary restrictions. needs and dietary restrictions.

Here are a few more diabetic-friendly main dish ideas:

Quinoa or brown rice bowls: Quinoa or brown rice bowls can be a delicious and healthy main dish. They can be paired with a variety of low-carb vegetables and topped with lean protein such as chicken or shrimp.

Lentil or bean-based stews: Lentil or bean-based stews can be a great source of fiber and protein. They can be made with a variety of low-carb vegetables such as carrots, celery, and tomatoes.

Turkey or chicken meatballs: Turkey or chicken meatballs can be a great source of lean protein. They can be paired with a variety of low-carb vegetables such as spaghetti squash or zucchini noodles.

Tofu or tempeh: Tofu or tempeh can be a great source of protein for diabetics. They can be grilled or stir-fried with a variety of low-carb vegetables such as bell peppers, onions, and broccoli.

It's important to note that having a balanced diet is essential for diabetic people, in order to maintain healthy blood sugar levels and reduce the risk of complications. It's essential to include a mix of different food groups in every meal, such as carbohydrates, proteins, and healthy fats. Additionally, it's crucial to consult with a ethereal provider or a registered dietitian to develop a personalized meal plan that fits your individual needs and dietary restrictions.

Here are a few diabetic-friendly dessert and sweet ideas

Fresh fruits: Fresh fruits such as berries, melons, and citrus fruits are naturally low in sugar and high in fiber and vitamins. They can be enjoyed on their own or topped with a dollop of low-fat whipped cream or yogurt.

Sorbet or frozen yogurt: Sorbet and frozen yogurt are lower in sugar than ice cream and can be a great option for diabetics.

Dark chocolate: Dark chocolate is high in antioxidants and can be a great option for diabetics in moderation.

Sugar-free jello or pudding: Jello and pudding made with sugar-free sweeteners can be a good option for diabetics.

Apple crisp: Apple crisp made with a topping of oats, nuts, and a small amount of butter or oil can be a good option for diabetics.

Lemon bars: Lemon bars made with a crust of almond flour or ground nuts and sweetened with a sugar substitute can be a good option for diabetics.

It's important to keep in mind that it's still important to watch portion sizes, even for diabetic-friendly desserts, and to consult with a ethereal provider or a registered dietitian to ensure that the desserts and sweets you choose are appropriate for your individual needs and dietary restrictions

Here are a few more diabetic-friendly dessert and sweet ideas:

Berries with Balsamic Vinegar: Berries such as strawberries, raspberries and blueberries can be a delicious, low-carb and sweet treat. They can be drizzled with balsamic vinegar, which adds a touch of sweetness and tanginess.

Chocolate Avocado Mousse: Avocados are high in healthy fats and fiber and can be used as a base for a rich and creamy chocolate mousse, sweetened with a sugar substitute.

Coconut Milk Panna Cotta: Panna cotta made with coconut milk and sweetened with a sugar substitute can be a delicious and healthy option for diabetics.

Sugar-free Cheesecake: Cheesecake made with sugar-free sweeteners and a crust made of nuts can be a good option for diabetics.

Flourless Chocolate Cake: This type of cakes are made with cocoa powder and ground nuts as a base, and sweetened with sugar substitutes. They are high in fiber, healthy fats, and lower in sugar than traditional cakes.

Chia seed pudding: Chia seed pudding is easy to make and it's a high-fiber, high-protein and low-carb dessert that can be sweetened with sugar substitutes or with natural sweeteners such as honey or maple syrup.

Again, it's important to be mindful of portion control and to consult with a ethereal provider or a registered dietitian.

A few diabetic-friendly beverage ideas

Water: Water is the best beverage choice for diabetics, as it is calorie-free and hydrating.

Unsweetened tea or coffee: Tea and coffee are naturally low in calories and sugar and can be enjoyed on their own or with a small amount of milk or a sugar substitute.

Unsweetened or sugar-free sparkling water: Sparkling water can be a refreshing option for diabetics, but it's important to choose a version that is unsweetened or sweetened with a sugar substitute.

Sugar-free or low-sugar sports drinks: Sports drinks can be a good option for diabetics who are engaging in intense physical activity, but it's important to choose a version that is low in sugar or sweetened with a sugar substitute.

Sugar-free or low-sugar herbal teas: Herbal teas such as mint, chamomile, and ginger are naturally low in calories and can be a relaxing and refreshing option for diabetics.

Dairy-free milk alternatives: Dairy-free milk alternatives such as almond milk, soy milk, and coconut milk can be a good option for diabetics, but it's important to choose versions that are unsweetened or sweetened with a sugar substitute.

It's important to consult with a ethereal provider

Here are a few diabetic-friendly beverage ideas

Water: Water is the best beverage choice for diabetics, as it is calorie-free and hydrating.

Unsweetened tea or coffee: Tea and coffee are naturally low in calories and sugar and can be enjoyed on their own or with a small amount of milk or a sugar substitute.

Unsweetened or sugar-free sparkling water: Sparkling water can be a refreshing option for diabetics, but it's important to choose a version that is unsweetened or sweetened with a sugar substitute.

Sugar-free or low-sugar sports drinks: Sports drinks can be a good option for diabetics who are engaging in intense physical activity, but it's important to choose a version that is low in sugar or sweetened with a sugar substitute.

Sugar-free or low-sugar herbal teas: Herbal teas such as mint, chamomile, and ginger are naturally low in calories and can be a relaxing and refreshing option for diabetics.

Dairy-free milk alternatives: Dairy-free milk alternatives such as almond milk, soy milk, and coconut milk can be a good option for diabetics, but it's important to choose versions that are unsweetened or sweetened with a sugar substitute.

It's important to consult with a ethereal provider

Here are a few more diabetic-friendly beverage ideas:

Vegetable juices: Vegetable juices such as carrot, beet, and cucumber juice can be a good option for diabetics as they are low in sugar and high in fiber and vitamins.

Low-carb protein shakes: Low-carb protein shakes can be a good option for diabetics as they provide a good source of protein and can be sweetened with a sugar substitute.

Kombucha: Kombucha is a fermented tea that is low in sugar and high in probiotics, it can be a good option for diabetics as a alternative for soda.

Coconut water: Coconut water is low in sugar and high in potassium, it can be a good alternative for sports drinks and it can help to replenish electrolytes.

Milk alternatives with low-carb sweeteners: there are many milk alternatives such as almond milk, soy milk, and coconut milk that are sweetened with low-carb sweeteners like Stevia and Erythritol.

It's important to note that even with diabetic-friendly beverages it's important to be mindful of portion sizes and to consult with a ethereal provider or a registered dietitian to ensure that the Eating out and traveling can be challenging for people with diabetes, but there are ways to make it easier to manage.

Tips for eating out and traveling with diabetes:

Plan advance: This will help you make a head: Before going out to eat or traveling, research the menu options and plan your meal choices in diabetes-friendly choices.

Ask for modifications: Don't be afraid to ask for modifications to menu items. For example, you can ask for your dish to be prepared without added sugar or oil, or ask for extra vegetables instead of rice or potatoes.

Watch portion sizes: When eating out or traveling, it can be easy to eat larger portions than you would at home. Be mindful of portion sizes and try to avoid overeating.

Bring your own snacks: When traveling, bring your own snacks such as nuts, seeds, or low-carb protein bars to help keep your blood sugar levels stable between meals.

Stay active: When traveling, try to incorporate physical activity into your day. This can be as simple as taking a walk or doing a workout in your hotel room.

Be prepared: When traveling it's important to be prepared for any situation, make sure you have a supply of your diabetes medication, a glucose meter, and any other necessary equipment.

Discuss with your ethereal provider: Before traveling or eating out, it's always best to consult with your ethereal provider or a certified diabetes educator to develop a plan that is safe and effective for you.

By following these tips, you can make eating out and traveling with diabetes easier to manage

and still enjoy your experiences. beverages you
choose are appropriate for your individual needs
and dietary restrictions.

Exercise

Exercise is an important part of managing diabetes. Regular physical activity can help control blood sugar levels, lower the risk of cardiovascular disease, and improve overall health. Here are a few ways that exercise can help manage diabetes:

Increases insulin sensitivity: Exercise can increase the body's sensitivity to insulin, which helps to lower blood sugar levels. This is particularly true for weight-bearing and high-intensity exercises.

Burns calories: Exercise burns calories, which can help with weight management. Maintaining a healthy weight is important for managing diabetes, as being overweight or obese can increase the risk of developing the disease.

Improves cardiovascular health: Exercise can improve cardiovascular health, which is important for people with diabetes as they have a higher risk of heart disease.

Reduces stress: Exercise can also help to reduce stress, which can be beneficial for managing diabetes as stress can cause blood sugar levels to spike.

Increases muscle mass: Exercise can increase muscle mass, which can help the body to use insulin more efficiently and lower blood sugar levels.

It's important to consult with a ethereal provider or a certified diabetes educator before starting an exercise program, as they can help to create a personalized exercise plan that is safe and effective for managing diabetes.

A combination of cardiovascular and strength training exercises is ideal for managing diabetes. Cardiovascular exercise such as walking, cycling, swimming, and dancing can help improve insulin sensitivity, burn calories, and improve cardiovascular health. Strength training exercises

such as weightlifting, resistance bands, and body
weight exercises can help increase muscle mass
and improve overall health.

types of exercises that are beneficial for managing diabetes.

Cardiovascular exercises: Cardiovascular exercises such as walking, running, cycling, swimming, and dancing are great for improving insulin sensitivity, burning calories, and improving cardiovascular health.

Strength training exercises: Strength training exercises such as weightlifting, resistance bands, and body weight exercises can help increase muscle mass, improve overall health, and improve insulin sensitivity.

Yoga and Pilates: Yoga and Pilates are great for improving flexibility, balance, and strength, and can also help to reduce stress and improve overall health.

High-Intensity Interval Training (HIIT): HIIT is a type of cardiovascular exercise that alternates between periods of high-intensity activity and recovery periods. It is great for burning calories and improve cardiovascular health, and can be done using body weight exercises, cycling, or running.

Tai chi: Tai chi is a low-impact martial art that combines movement and breathing. It is great for improving balance, flexibility and muscle strength and it also helps to reduce stress and improve overall health.

It's important to consult with a ethereal provider or a certified diabetes educator before starting an exercise program, as they can help to create a personalized exercise plan that is safe and effective.

Managing diabetes with medications and how it affects the body

Here are a few details on the medications used to manage diabetes and their potential advantages and side effects:

Insulin: Insulin is a hormone that helps to regulate blood sugar levels. It is effective in controlling blood sugar levels in people with type 1 diabetes and some with type 2 diabetes. Advantages include its effectiveness and its ability to mimic the body's natural insulin production. Common side effects include low blood sugar, weight gain, and injection site reactions.

Metformin: Metformin is a medication that helps to lower blood sugar levels by reducing the amount of glucose produced by the liver and increasing the sensitivity of cells to insulin. Advantages include it's effectiveness, and it's relatively low cost. Common side effects include stomach upset, diarrhea and metallic taste in mouth.

Sulfonylureas: Sulfonylureas are a class of medications that help to lower blood sugar levels by increasing the amount of insulin produced by the pancreas. Advantages include effectiveness in controlling blood sugar levels and relatively low cost. Common side effects include weight gain, low blood sugar, and stomach upset.

DPP-4 inhibitors: DPP-4 inhibitors are a class of medications that help to lower blood sugar levels by increasing the amount of incretin hormones in the body. Advantages include effectiveness in controlling blood sugar levels and relatively low risk of low blood sugar. Common side effects include stomach upset, diarrhea, and upper respiratory tract infections.

GLP-1 receptor agonists: GLP-1 receptor agonists are a class of medications that help to lower blood sugar levels by increasing the amount of incretin hormones in the body. Advantages include effectiveness in controlling blood sugar levels and weight loss. Common side effects include nausea, diarrhea, and stomach upset.

SGLT2 inhibitors:anaging diabetes.

Continuous Glucose Monitoring (CGM) is a technology that allows people with diabetes to track their blood sugar levels in real-time. It involves wearing a small sensor under the skin that continuously measures glucose levels in the fluid under the skin. The sensor is connected to a small device that displays the glucose level and trends, and can alert the person if their glucose level is too high or too low.
CGM can be especially beneficial for people with type 1 diabetes and people with type 2 diabetes who use insulin. Here are a few ways that CGM can help manage diabetes:

Real-time glucose monitoring: CGM allows for continuous monitoring of glucose levels, providing a more complete picture of blood sugar patterns. This can help dosing, food choices, and physically active people with diabetes make more informed decisions about insulin.

Alerts for high and low glucose levels: CGM devices can alert the person if their glucose level is too high or too low, allowing them to take corrective action before a problem becomes severe.

Trend analysis: CGM devices can provide trend analysis, which can help people with diabetes and their ethereal providers identify patterns and areas that need improvement.

Fewer finger pricks: CGM eliminates the need for frequent finger pricks to check blood sugar levels, which can be uncomfortable and inconvenient.

Better A1C control: A1C is a measure of average blood sugar levels over the past 2-3 months, and it is a key indicator of diabetes control. CGM can help people with diabetes achieve better A1C control by providing more accurate and frequent glucose measurements.

It's important to note that CGM is not suitable for everyone, and it's important to consult with a ethereal provider or a certified diabetes educator to determine if CGM is appropriate for you and h-Insulin pumps are small, computerized devices that deliver insulin to the body through a small tube, called a catheter, that is inserted under the skin. Insulin pumps can be an effective tool for managing diabetes, especially for people with type 1 diabetes who need to take multiple doses of insulin daily.

ways that insulin pumps can help manage diabetes:

More precise insulin dosing: Insulin pumps allow for more precise insulin dosing, which can help to better control blood sugar levels.

Basal rate adjustments: Insulin pumps allow for basal rate adjustments, which are small adjustments to the insulin dosage given continuously throughout the day to maintain a steady blood sugar level.

Bolus adjustments: Insulin pumps allow for bolus adjustments, which are adjustments to the insulin dosage given before or after a meal to account for the glucose from the food.

Better flexibility: Insulin pumps offer more flexibility for people with diabetes, as they can be worn discreetly under clothing and allow for more freedom in meal times and physical activity.

Continuous glucose monitoring: Some insulin pumps can be integrated with continuous glucose monitoring (CGM) systems, allowing for even more accurate insulin dosing and glucose management.

Reduced risk of hypoglycemia: Insulin pumps can reduce the risk of hypoglycemia (low blood sugar) by providing more precise insulin dosing and by allowing for adjustments to insulin dosage in real-time.

It's important to note that insulin pumps are not suitable for everyone and it's important to consult with a ethereal provider or a certified diabetes educator to determine if an insulin pump is appropriate for you, and to learn how to properly use it.

understand the results of your A1C test, and to determine how often it should be repeated.

Ways that A1C test can help manage diabetes:

Setting goals: A1C test results can be used to set goals for blood sugar control. For example, if your A1C level is high, your ethereal provider may recommend that you aim to lower it by a certain percentage over the next few months.

Evaluating treatment effectiveness: A1C test results can be used to evaluate the effectiveness of diabetes treatment. For example, if your A1C level decreases after starting a new medication or making changes to your diet and exercise routine, it may indicate that the treatment is working well.

Identifying uncontrolled diabetes: A1C test results can be used to identify uncontrolled diabetes. If A1C test results are consistently above the recommended level, it may indicate that the current treatment plan is not working effectively and adjustments may need to be made.

Identifying prediabetes: A1C test results can be used to identify prediabetes, which is a condition in which blood sugar levels are higher than normal but not yet high enough to be diagnosed as diabetes. Identifying prediabetes early can help prevent or delay the development of diabetes.

It's important to note that A1C test should be done in conjunction with other diabetes tests, such as fasting glucose tests, oral glucose tolerance tests, and daily glucose monitoring. It's also important to consult with a ethereal provider or a certified diabetes educator to understand the results of your A1C test and to determine how often it should be repeated.

An A1C test, also known as a glycated hemoglobin test, is a blood test that measures the average blood sugar level over the past 2-3 months. It is a key indicator of diabetes control and can be used to monitor the effectiveness of diabetes management. The test is often used to diagnose diabetes and to monitor the effectiveness of treatment for people with diabetes.

A1C test results are expressed as a percentage, with higher values indicating higher blood sugar levels. The American Diabetes Association (ADA) recommends that people with diabetes aim for an A1C level of less than 7%.

ways that A1C tests can help manage diabetes

Diagnosis of diabetes: A1C tests are often used to diagnose diabetes, as they can provide a clear picture of blood sugar control over the past 2-3 months.

Monitoring diabetes control: A1C tests can be used to monitor diabetes control over time, allowing people with diabetes and their ethereal providers to see if the treatment plan is working and to make adjustments as needed.

Identifying trends: A1C tests can help identify trends in blood sugar control, which can help people with diabetes and their ethereal providers identify areas that need improvement.

Predicting complications: A1C tests can be used to predict the risk of complications related to diabetes, such as heart disease and kidney disease.

Infrequent testing: A1C tests don't need to be done as frequently as other diabetes tests, such as daily glucose monitoring, making it more convenient for people with diabetes.

It is important to note that A1C test results can be influenced by factors such as iron deficiency anemia, and kidney or liver disease. It's important to consult with a ethereal provider or a certified diabetes educator to understand the results of your A1C test, and to determine how often it should be repeated.

Managing psychological and emotional aspects of living with diabetes

Living with diabetes can have significant psychological and emotional impacts on a person's life. It is important to manage these aspects of diabetes to maintain overall health and well-being. Here are some tips for managing the psychological and emotional aspects of living with diabetes:

Acceptance: Accepting the diagnosis and understanding the realities of living with diabetes is an important step in managing the emotional side of diabetes.

Support network: Surround yourself with a support network of family and friends who understand what you're going through and can offer encouragement and support. Joining a diabetes support group can also be helpful.

Healthy coping mechanisms: Finding healthy ways to cope with stress, such as exercise, mindfulness, and counseling, can help manage the emotional impact of diabetes.

Good self-care: Taking care of oneself through healthy eating, regular exercise, and good sleep habits can help manage stress levels and improve overall well-being.

Open communication: Talking openly and honestly with your healthcare team about any emotional or psychological concerns can help ensure that they are addressed and treated appropriately.

Positive outlook: Focusing on the positive aspects of life and finding joy and purpose in daily activities can help maintain a positive outlook and improve overall well-being.

Remember, everyone reacts differently to a diabetes diagnosis, and it is important to be patient with oneself and seek help when needed. With the right support and strategies in place, it is possible to manage the psychological and emotional aspects of living with diabetes and live a fulfilling life.

Some testimonies of people diagnosed with the disease

Here are some detailed success stories of individuals with diabetes who have overcome challenges and found success and happiness:

Halle Berry: Halle Berry was diagnosed with type 1 diabetes at the age of 22 and was initially devastated by the news. She faced challenges with managing her blood sugar levels and felt limited by her condition. Despite these challenges, Halle was able to find success in her personal and professional life by managing her diabetes effectively. She has become a Hollywood icon and an advocate for diabetes education and awareness. Halle credits her success to a healthy diet, regular exercise, and careful monitoring of her blood sugar levels.

Novak Djokovic: Novak Djokovic, a world-renowned tennis player, was diagnosed with type 1 diabetes at the age of 18. Despite the challenges, Novak was able to find success in his tennis career by managing his diabetes effectively. He closely monitors his blood sugar levels and adjusts his insulin dosage as needed. Novak also follows a healthy diet and exercises regularly to maintain his physical fitness and support his diabetes management. He credits his success to his determination, hard work, and commitment to his health.

Salma Hayek: Salma Hayek was diagnosed with gestational diabetes during her pregnancy and was initially frightened by the news. She faced challenges with managing her blood sugar levels and adjusting to a new diet and lifestyle. Despite these challenges, Salma was able to successfully manage her diabetes and give birth to a healthy baby. She has since become an advocate for healthy eating and diabetes management. Salma encourages others to make healthy food choices and find joy in the process of eating well. She also encourages individuals with diabetes to seek support from their healthcare team and find the resources they need to succeed.

Mary Tyler Moore: Mary Tyler Moore was diagnosed with type 1 diabetes at the age of 33 and faced challenges with managing her blood sugar levels and adjusting to a new diet and lifestyle. Despite these challenges, Mary was able to find success in her personal and professional life by managing her diabetes effectively. She was a strong advocate for diabetes education and awareness and encouraged others with diabetes to take control of their health. Mary was committed to her health and made lifestyle changes to support her diabetes management. She found success and happiness in her personal and professional life and inspired others with diabetes to do the same.

David Pearson: David Pearson, a former NASCAR driver, was diagnosed with type 2 diabetes in his later years. Despite the challenges, David was able to find success in his personal life by managing his diabetes effectively. He made lifestyle changes such as adopting a healthy diet, increasing his physical activity, and quitting smoking. David was committed to his health and monitored his blood sugar levels regularly. He encouraged others with diabetes to take control of their health and make lifestyle changes to support their diabetes management. David found happiness and fulfillment in his later years and inspired others with diabetes to do the same.

These success stories demonstrate that individuals with diabetes can overcome challenges and find success and happiness by effectively managing their condition. By taking control of their health, making lifestyle changes, and seeking support from their healthcare team, individuals with diabetes can live their best lives. These stories provide encouragement and inspiration for individuals with diabetes and demonstrate the potential for a healthy and fulfilling life with diabetes.

Conclusion

Managing diabetes can be a complex and ongoing process. It involves monitoring blood sugar levels, making healthy lifestyle choices, taking medications as prescribed, and working closely with a health-care provider or certified diabetes educator.

major key strategies for managing diabetes include:

Eating a healthy, balanced diet

Engaging in regular physical activity

Monitoring blood sugar levels regularly

Taking medications as prescribed

Monitoring blood pressure and cholesterol levels

Keeping regular follow-up appointments with a health-care provider

Managing stress

In addition to these strategies, there are many resources available to help people with diabetes manage their condition. These resources include:

American Diabetes Association (ADA)

American Association of Diabetes Educators (AADE)

International Diabetes Federation (IDF)

Juvenile Diabetes Research Foundation (JDRF)

National Institute of Diabetes and Digestive and Kidney Diseases (NIDDK)

These organizations offer a wealth of information on diabetes management, including information on healthy eating, physical activity, medications, and diabetes complications. They also offer support and resources for people with diabetes and their families.

It is also important to have a support system, whether it be a family member or friend, someone who is going through the same thing as you, or a support group. This is a great way to share experiences, get advice and ask questions.

It is also important to talk to your ethereal provider or certified diabetes educator about any questions or concerns you may have about managing your diabetes. They can provide you with the guidance and support you need to effectively manage your condition and live a healthy, fulfilling life.